CW0470331

RENAL DIET COOKBOOK:

A Simple And Easy Guide To 50 Low-Sodium, Potassium And Phosphorus Recipes From Breakfast To Desserts. Learn How To Manage Your Kidney Disease And Avoid Dialysis.

Susan Johnson

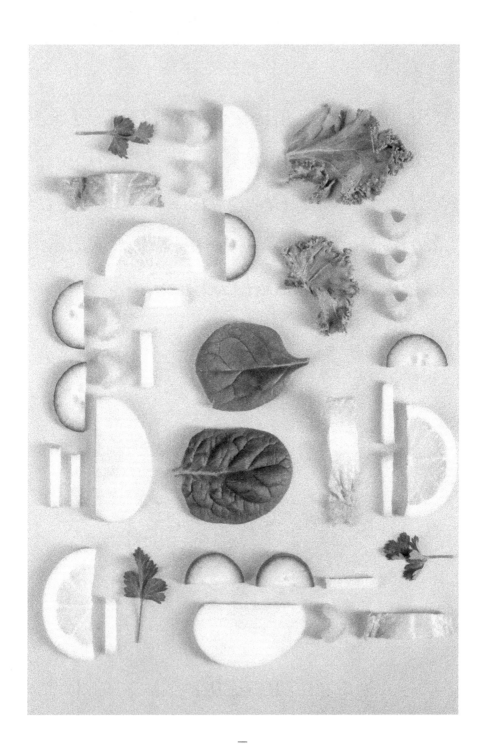

The information in the following pages is broadly considered a truthful and accurate account of facts and as such, any inattention, use, or misuse of the information in question by the reader will render any resulting actions solely under their purview. There are no scenarios in which the publisher or the original author of this work can be in any fashion deemed liable for any hardship or damages that may befall them after undertaking information described herein.

Additionally, the information in the following pages is intended only for informational purposes and should thus be thought of as universal. As befitting its nature, it is presented without assurance regarding its prolonged validity or interim quality. Trademarks that are mentioned are done without written consent and can in no way be considered an endorsement from the trademark holder.

Table of contents

—

Introduction

When we follow the renal diet, we will make use of all the information about various components and minerals of foods to prepare a meal that is as ideal for our body as possible. One of the renal diet's main aims is to manage sodium, potassium, and phosphorus intake. Simultaneously, the renal diet focuses on consuming high-quality protein and limiting the consumption of fluids. Knowing about what you should eat and what you shouldn't go a long way in finding out if there is anything in particular that you should avoid (due to allergies, for example).

So how exactly does the renal diet benefit you?

Preventing Diabetes and High Blood Pressure from Worsening

When you manage two of the biggest contributors of CKD, you are greatly delaying the effects of the disease. You are getting out of a loop where either diabetes or high blood pressure makes the disease worse, further worsening either of the two conditions, which results in the disease entering a worse phase, and on it goes. This loop continues until it results in complete kidney failure.

Provides Essential Nutrients

The renal diet includes a lot of the good stuff and removes as much unnecessary stuff as possible. This means that the diet uses select ingredients to give you many vital nutrients in one meal. The diet's ability to filter through various kinds of food to produce something extremely healthy for you is why it is popular among people with CKD. They simply want to minimize the consumption of certain minerals.

Good Energy

One of the thoughts that zip through people's minds (I say 'zip' because it usually does not stay too long, and you will find out why) is if they might receive the right about of energy from a renal diet. We are all used to consuming a certain type of food that includes numerous minerals and essential components. The renal diet is going to cut many of those components out of your diet. It's like looking at a five-story building, deciding that the top three stories don't matter, and just decided to bulldoze the unwanted floors! Indeed, a renal diet will feel like an extreme diet since you are going to cut down on a lot of foods suddenly. You are going to 'bulldoze' them from your daily meals.

However, with the kind of food you are going to eat, you won't have to worry about energy. When you are on a renal diet, you can perform many physical activities that you might have thought you wouldn't be able to engage in after entering the diet.

You will get your energy from so many healthy and nutritious sources, as you will discover once you start reading through the recipes.

Should you choose to accept it, your mission is to ensure that you minimize waste buildup in your kidneys. To do that, you need to watch what you eat, carefully preparing or arranging your meals so that you receive the required nutrition, minus all the unnecessary components.

This is where a renal diet becomes an essential component of your life.

Before delving deeper into the diet itself, let us look at some of the important substances that people with CKD need to manage.

Sodium

Suppose you have been enjoying your pasta, nachos, pizzas, juicy steaks, lip-smacking' burgers, or practically any of your favorite savory food items. In that case, the chances are that you have been consuming sodium.

Why? Well, this mineral is commonly found in salt. Whether you use table salt or sea salt, you are going to find sodium in them.

If you have heard people claim that sodium is harmful to your body, let me tell you that it is not entirely true. We need sodium in our bodies. The mineral helps our body maintain a balance in the levels of water within and around our cells. At the same time, it also maintains your blood pressure levels.

Surprised? You might have thought that sodium makes things worse, but there is a medical condition called hypernatremia, or "low blood sodium." When sodium levels drop to a low enough level, then you experience all the symptoms below:

- weakness
- nausea
- vomiting
- fatigue or low energy
- headache
- irritability
- muscle cramps or spasms
- confusion

In conclusion, sodium is essential for your body. But when you are on a renal diet, you control the amount of salt that you add to your food. Since the kidneys are rather sensitive at this point, there is no need to exacerbate their condition by adding more sodium.

This might prove difficult for people since they are used to having salt as a flavoring ingredient in their foods. But that is why we will use recipes full of flavors that you will enjoy (more on that when we get started on the recipes).

Potassium

Apart from regulating fluids in the body, it also aids the body in passing messages between the body and the brain. Like sodium, potassium is classified as an electrolyte, a term used to refer to a family of minerals that react in water. When potassium is dissolved in water, it produces positively charged ions. Using these ions, potassium can conduct electricity, which allows it to carry out some incredibly important functions. Take, for example, the messages that are communicated between the brain and the body. These messages are sent back and forth in the form of impulses. But one has to wonder; what exactly creates those impulses? It's not like our body has an inbuilt electrical generator.

The answer lies in the ions. We have already established that sodium and potassium are both electrolytes and produce ions. The impulses are created when sodium ions move into the cells, and potassium ions move out of the cell. This movement changes the voltage of the cell, producing impulses. The way the impulses are created is similar to Morse code but takes place much faster (it has to for your body to react, manage processes, or perform tasks). When the level of potassium falls, the body's ability to generate nerve impulses gets affected.

Wait a minute. So potassium is good. Does that mean I am asking you to let your body give up on normal nerve impulses to keep your kidneys safe? Is that the only choice? That's a tough choice to make!

More specifically, they could change the heartbeats' rhythm, which could lead to a potential heart attack. But don't worry. This does not happen with just a mild increase in potassium. There has to be a significant increase to cause such a devastating result.

Nevertheless, we are going to avoid even reaching a 'mild' increase. I placed the mild in quotes because there is no actual benchmark to gauge if the potassium content in your blood is mild or potentially life-threatening. It all depends on various factors in the body. I shall list down a few foods that are high in potassium that you should watch out for:

- Melons such as cantaloupe and honeydew (watermelon is acceptable)
- Oranges and orange juice
- Winter squash

- Pumpkin
- Bananas
- Prune juice
- Grapefruit juice
- Dried beans – all kinds

Try to avoid granola bars (even though they are advertised as nutritious) and bran cereals.

Phosphorus

Finally, we have phosphorus. This mineral makes up about 1% of your body weight. That may not seem like a lot in actuality, but remember that our body consists of a lot of water. For this reason, oxygen makes up 62% of our total body weight, followed by carbon at 18%, hydrogen at 9%, and nitrogen at 3%. But guess which are the next two major elements in the human body?

Calcium at 1.5%.

Phosphorus at 1%.

So you see, even though phosphorus makes up just 1% of the total body weight, it is still a significant element.

What is it used for?

Let me put it this way. Phosphorus is one of the reasons that you can smile wide. It is the reason your skin and other parts of the body are the way they are and do not just fall on the floor, like the way a piece of cloth might when you drop it. Phosphorus is responsible for forming your teeth and the bones that keep your body structure the way it currently is.

Pretty fantastic, isn't it? We often nominate calcium as the main element in the formation of teeth and bones but forget the less popular and often overlooked partner element that helps with the same task.

However, the fact that phosphorus keeps our teeth and bones healthy is something people eventually discover. They don't discover that phosphorus also plays an important role in helping the body use fats and carbohydrates. The mineral is truly important for the everyday function of the body.

When kidney problems strike us, we don't need the extra amount of phosphorus. While phosphorus is truly important for our bones and teeth, an excessive amount in the blood can lead to weaker bones. Since most of the food that we eat already includes phosphorus, we will try and avoid anything that has a high percentage of the mineral.

Fluids

Water sustains us. After all, 60% of the human adult's body is composed of water. This is why you might have heard of popular recommendations on how you should be having about eight glasses of water per day.

There is still a debate on exactly how much water is needed by an individual daily. But the fact remains; we need enough to avoid dehydration and keep the body functioning normally.

When you have kidney disease, you may not need as much fluid as you did before. This is because damaged kidneys do not dispose of extra fluids as well as they should. All the extra fluid in your body could be dangerous. It could cause swelling in various areas, high blood pressure, and heart problems. Fluid can also build up around your lungs, preventing you from breathing normally.

There is no measurement of how much fluid is considered as extra fluid. I strongly suggest that you should visit the doctor and get more information about fluid retention from him or her. The doctor will guide you better and help you understand how much fluids you might require. The thing to understand here is that many of the foods that we eat, including fruits, vegetables, and most soups, have water content in them as well. Getting to know your kidney's ability to hold on to fluids will help you prepare or plan better meals for yourself.

Chapter 1. Breakfast

1. Overnight Oats Three Ways

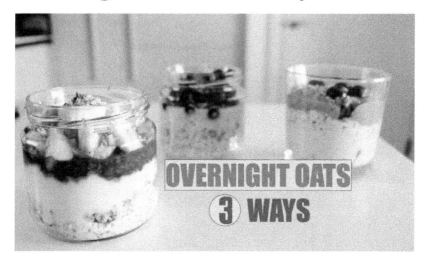

Preparation Time: 5 minutes

Cooking Time: 5 minutes

Servings: 2 servings

Ingredients:

- ¾ cup or unsweetened store-bought rice milk

- ½ cup plain, unsweetened yogurt

- ½ cup rolled oats

- 1 tablespoon ground flaxseed

- 1 teaspoon vanilla extract

- 2 teaspoons honey

Directions:

1. In a bowl, combine the rice milk, yogurt, oats, flaxseed, vanilla, and honey.

2. Add the ingredients to make your preferred variation, and stir to blend.

3. Divide between two jars, cover, and refrigerate for at least 4 hours or overnight.

Nutrition: Calories: 196; Total Fat: 7g; Saturated Fat: 2g; Cholesterol: 7mg; Carbohydrates: 25g; Fiber: 3g; Protein: 8g; Phosphorus: 99mg; Potassium: 114mg; Sodium: 63mg

2. Buckwheat Pancakes

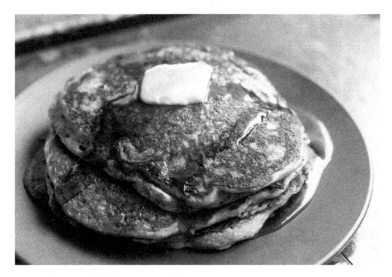

Preparation Time: 10 minutes

Cooking Time: 15 minutes

Servings: 4 servings

Ingredients:

- 1¾ cups or unsweetened store-bought rice milk

- 2 teaspoons white vinegar

- 1 cup buckwheat flour

- ½ cup all-purpose flour

- 1 tablespoon sugar

- 1 large egg

- 2 teaspoons Phosphorus-Free baking powder

- 1 teaspoon vanilla extract

- 2 tablespoons butter, for the skillet

Directions:

1. Mix the rice milk and vinegar. Let sit for 10 minutes.

2. Combine the buckwheat flour and all-purpose flour in a bowl

3. Add the sugar and baking powder.

4. Add the ingredients to the dry, and mix until just mixed.

5. Cook for 2 to 3 minutes, until small bubbles form on the surface of the pancakes.

6. Handover the pancakes to a serving platter, and in batches, continue cooking the remaining batter in the skillet, adding more butter as needed.

Nutrition: Calories: 264; Total Fat: 9g; Saturated Fat: 3g; Cholesterol: 58mg; Carbohydrates: 39g; Fiber: 3g; Protein: 7g; Phosphorus: 147mg; Potassium: 399mg; Sodium: 232mg

3. Avocado Egg Bake

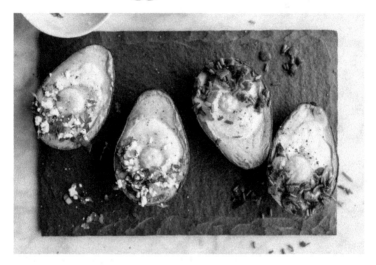

Preparation Time: 5 minutes

Cooking Time: 15 minutes

Servings: 2 servings

Ingredients:

- 1 avocado, halved

- 2 large eggs

- Freshly ground black pepper

- 1 tablespoon chopped parsley

Directions:

1. Beat 1 egg carefully

2. place the avocado halves cut-side up on baking sheet

3. Transfer the egg into one half.

4. Repeat with the next egg and avocado half. Season with pepper.

5. Bake for 15 minutes, until the egg is set.

Nutrition: Calories: 242; Total Fat: 20g; Saturated Fat: 4g; Cholesterol: 208mg; Carbohydrates: 9g; Fiber: 7g; Protein: 9g; Phosphorus: 164mg; Potassium: 575mg; Sodium: 88mg

4. Broccoli Basil Quiche

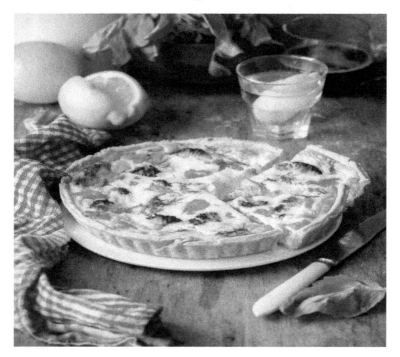

Preparation Time: 10 minutes

Cooking Time: 55 minutes

Servings: 8 servings

Ingredients:

- 1 store-bought frozen piecrust

- 2 cups finely chopped broccoli

- 1 tomato, chopped

- 2 scallions, chopped

- 3 eggs, beaten

- 2 tablespoons chopped basil

- 1 cup or unsweetened store-bought rice milk

- ½ cup crumbled feta cheese

- 1 garlic clove, minced

- 1 tablespoon all-purpose flour

- Freshly ground black pepper

Directions:

1. Preheat the oven to 450°F.

2. Line a pie pan with the piecrust, and use a fork to pierce the crust in several places.

3. Bake the crust for 10 minutes. Remove from the oven and reduce the temperature to 325°F.

4. combine the broccoli, tomato, scallions, eggs, basil, rice milk, feta, garlic, and flour. Season with pepper.

5. Pour the broccoli-and-egg mixture into the prepared pie pan.

6. Bake for 35 to 45 minutes, until a knife inserted in the center comes out clean.

Nutrition: Calories: 160; Total Fat: 10g; Saturated Fat: 3g; Cholesterol: 87mg; Carbohydrates: 13g; Fiber: 1g; Protein: 6g; Phosphorus: 101mg; Potassium: 173mg; Sodium: 259mg

5. Berry Chia with Yogurt

Preparation Time: 35 minutes

Cooking time: 5 minutes

Servings:4

Ingredients:

- ½ cup chia seeds, dried

- 2 cup Plain yogurt

- 1/3 cup strawberries, chopped

- ¼ cup blackberries

- ¼ cup raspberries

- 4 teaspoons Splenda

Directions:

1. Mix up together Plain yogurt with Splenda, and chia seeds.

2. Transfer the mixture into the serving ramekins (jars) and leave for 35 minutes.

3. After this, add blackberries, raspberries, and strawberries. Mix up the meal well.

Nutrition:

calories 257,

fat 10.3,

fiber 11,

carbs 27.2,

protein 12

6. Arugula Eggs with Chili Peppers

Preparation Time: 7 minutes

Cooking time: 10 minutes

Servings: 4

Ingredients:

- 2 cups arugula, chopped

- 3 eggs, beaten

- ½ chili pepper, chopped

- 1 tablespoon butter

- 1 oz. Parmesan, grated

Directions:

1. Toss butter in the skillet and melt it.

2. Add arugula and sauté it over the medium heat for 5 minutes. Stir it from time to time.

3. Meanwhile, mix up together Parmesan, chili pepper, and eggs.

4. Pour the egg mixture over the arugula and scramble well.

5. Cook the breakfast for 5 minutes more over the medium heat.

Nutrition:

calories 98,

fat 7.8,

fiber 0.2,

carbs 0.9,

protein 6.7

7. Breakfast Skillet

Preparation Time: 7 minutes

Cooking time: 25 minutes

Servings: 5

Ingredients:

- 1 cup cauliflower, chopped

- 1 tablespoon olive oil

- ½ red onion, diced

- 1 tablespoon Plain yogurt

- ½ teaspoon ground black pepper

- 1 teaspoon dried cilantro

- 1 teaspoon dried oregano

- 1 bell pepper, chopped

- 1/3 cup milk

- ½ teaspoon Za'atar

- 1 tablespoon lemon juice

- 1 russet potato, chopped

Directions:

1. Pour olive oil in the skillet and preheat it.

2. Add chopped russet potato and roast it for 5 minutes.

3. After this, add cauliflower, ground black pepper, cilantro, oregano, and bell pepper.

4. Roast the mixture for 10 minutes over the medium heat.

5. Then add milk, Za'atar, and Plain Yogurt. Stir it well.

6. Sauté the mixture 10 minutes.

7. Top the cooked meal with diced red onion and sprinkle with lemon juice.

8. It is recommended to serve the breakfast hot.

Nutrition:

calories 112,

fat 3.4,

fiber 2.6,

carbs 18.1,

protein 3.1

8. Eggplant Chicken Sandwich

Preparation Time: 10 minutes

Cooking time: 15 minutes

Servings: 2

Ingredients:

- 1 eggplant, trimmed

- 10 oz. chicken fillet

- 1 teaspoon Plain yogurt

- ½ teaspoon minced garlic

- 1 tablespoon fresh cilantro, chopped

- 2 lettuce leaves

- 1 teaspoon olive oil

- ½ teaspoon salt

- ½ teaspoon chili pepper

- 1 teaspoon butter

Directions:

1. Slice the eggplant lengthwise into 4 slices.

2. Rub the eggplant slices with minced garlic and brush with olive oil.

3. Grill the eggplant slices on the preheated to 375F grill for 3 minutes from each side.

4. Meanwhile, rub the chicken fillet with salt and chili pepper.

5. Place it in the skillet and add butter.

6. Roast the chicken for 6 minutes from each side over the medium-high heat.

7. Cool the cooked eggplants gently and spread one side of them with Plain yogurt.

8. Add lettuce leaves and chopped fresh cilantro.

9. After this, slice the cooked chicken fillet and add over the lettuce.

10. Cover it with the remaining sliced eggplant to get the sandwich shape. Pin the sandwich with the toothpick if needed.

Nutrition:

calories 368,

fat 15.2,

fiber 8.2,

carbs 14.2,

protein 43.5

9. Panzanella Salad

Preparation Time: 10 minutes

Cooking time: 5 minutes

Servings: 4

Ingredients:

- 3 tomatoes, chopped

- 2 cucumbers, chopped

- 1 red onion, sliced

- 2 red bell peppers, chopped

- ¼ cup fresh cilantro, chopped

- 1 tablespoon capers

- 1 oz. whole-grain bread, chopped

- 1 tablespoon canola oil

- ½ teaspoon minced garlic

- 1 tablespoon Dijon mustard

- 1 teaspoon olive oil

- 1 teaspoon lime juice

Directions:

1. Pour canola oil in the skillet and bring it to boil.

2. Add chopped bread and roast it until crunchy (3-5 minutes).

3. Meanwhile, in the salad bowl combine sliced red onion, cucumbers, tomatoes, bell peppers, cilantro, capers, and mix up gently.

4. Make the dressing: mix up together lime juice, olive oil, Dijon mustard, and minced garlic.

5. Transfer the dressing over the salad and stir it directly before serving.

Nutrition:

calories 136,

fat 5.7,

fiber 4.1,

carbs 20.2,

protein 4.1

10.   Shrimp Bruschetta

Preparation Time: 15 minutes

Cooking time: 10 minutes

Servings: 4

Ingredients:

- 13 oz. shrimps, peeled

- 1 tablespoon tomato sauce

- ½ teaspoon Splenda

- ¼ teaspoon garlic powder

- 1 teaspoon fresh parsley, chopped

- ½ teaspoon olive oil

- 1 teaspoon lemon juice

- 4 whole-grain bread slices

- 1 cup water, for cooking

Directions:

1. Transfer water in the saucepan and bring it to boil.

2. Add shrimps and boil them over the high heat for 5 minutes.

3. After this, drain shrimps and chill them to the room temperature.

4. Mix up together shrimps with Splenda, garlic powder, tomato sauce, and fresh parsley.

5. Add lemon juice and stir gently.

6. Preheat the oven to 360F.

7. Put the bread slices with olive oil and bake for 3 minutes.

8. Then place the shrimp mixture on the bread. Bruschetta is cooked.

Nutrition:

calories 199,

fat 3.7,

fiber 2.1,

carbs 15.3,

protein 24.1

11. Strawberry Muesli

Preparation Time: 10 minutes

Cooking time: 30 minutes

Servings: 4

Ingredients:

2 cups Greek yogurt

1 ½ cup strawberries, sliced

1 ½ cup Muesli

4 teaspoon maple syrup

¾ teaspoon ground cinnamon

Directions:

Put Greek yogurt in the food processor.

Add 1 cup of strawberries, maple syrup, and ground cinnamon.

Blend the ingredients until you get smooth mass.

Transfer the yogurt mass in the serving bowls.

Add Muesli and stir well.

Leave the meal for 30 minutes in the fridge.

After this, decorate it with remaining sliced strawberries.

Nutrition:

calories 149,

fat 2.6,

fiber 3.6,

carbs 21.6,

protein 12

12.   Yogurt Bulgur

Preparation Time: 10 minutes

Cooking time: 15 minutes

Servings: 3

Ingredients:

- 1 cup bulgur

- 2 cups Greek yogurt

- 1 ½ cup water

- ½ teaspoon salt

- 1 teaspoon olive oil

Directions:

1. Pour olive oil in the saucepan and add bulgur.

2. Roast it over the medium heat for 2-3 minutes. Stir it from time to time.

3. After this, add salt and water.

4. Close the lid and cook bulgur for 15 minutes over the medium heat.

5. Then chill the cooked bulgur well and combine it with Greek yogurt. Stir it carefully.

6. Transfer the cooked meal into the serving plates. The yogurt bulgur tastes the best when it is cold.

Nutrition:

calories 274,

fat 4.9,

fiber 8.5,

carbs 40.8,

protein 19.2

13.   Chia Pudding

Preparation Time: 10 minutes

Cooking time: 30 minutes

Servings: 2

Ingredients:

- ½ cup raspberries

- 2 teaspoons maple syrup

- 1 ½ cup Plain yogurt

- ¼ teaspoon ground cardamom

- 1/3 cup Chia seeds, dried

Directions:

1. Mix up together Plain yogurt with maple syrup and ground cardamom.

2. Add Chia seeds. Stir it gently.

3. Put the yogurt in the serving glasses and top with the raspberries.

4. Refrigerate the breakfast for at least 30 minutes or overnight.

Nutrition:

calories 303,

fat 11.2,

fiber 11.8,

carbs 33.2,

protein 15.5

Chapter 2. Main Dishes

14.   Tofu Hoisin Sauté

Preparation Time: 15 minutes

Cooking Time: 20 minutes

Servings: 4

Ingredients:

2 tablespoons of hoisin sauce

2 tablespoons of rice vinegar

1 teaspoon of cornstarch

2 tablespoons of olive oil

1 (15-ounce) package extra-firm tofu, cut into 1-inch cubes

2 cups of unpeeled cubed eggplant

2 scallions, white and green parts, sliced

2 teaspoons of minced garlic

1 jalapeño pepper, minced

2 tablespoons of chopped fresh cilantro

Directions:

In a small bowl, whisk together the hoisin sauce, rice vinegar, and cornstarch.

Heat the olive oil in pan.

Add the tofu, and sauté gently until golden brown, about 10 minutes, and transfer to a plate.

Reduce the heat to medium. Add the eggplant, scallions, garlic, jalapeño pepper, and sauté until tender and fragrant, about 6 minutes.

Stir in the reserved sauce, and toss until the sauce thickens about 2 minutes. Stir in the tofu and cilantro, and serve hot.

Low-sodium tip Hoisin sauce is made with soy sauce, containing a hefty amount of sodium per serving. This recipe would still be tasty, while slightly less intensely flavored if you use 1 tablespoon of hoisin sauce instead of 2 tablespoons.

Nutrition:

Calories: 105

Total fat: 4g

Saturated fat: 1g

Cholesterol: 0mg

Sodium: 234mg

Carbohydrates: 9g

Fiber: 2g

Phosphorus: 105mg

Potassium: 192mg

Protein: 8g

15.   Sweet Potato Curry

Preparation Time: 20 minutes

Cooking Time: 20 minutes

Servings: 6

Ingredients:

2 teaspoons of olive oil

1 medium sweet onion, chopped

1 tablespoon of grated peeled fresh ginger

1 teaspoon of minced fresh garlic

2 cups of diced peeled sweet potatoes

1 cup of diced carrots

1 cup of water

½ cup of heavy (whipping) cream

1 tablespoon of curry powder

1 teaspoon of ground cumin

2 tablespoons of low-fat plain yogurt

2 tablespoons of chopped fresh cilantro

Directions:

In a saucepan, heat the olive oil.

Add the onion, ginger, and garlic and sauté until softened, about 3 minutes.

Add the sweet potatoes, carrots, water, cream, curry powder, and cumin and stir to mix well. Bring the mixture to a boil.

Lessening the heat to low, and simmer until the vegetables are tender, about 15 minutes.

Serve immediately, topped with the yogurt and cilantro.

Nutrition:

Calories: 132

Total fat: 9g

Saturated fat: 5g

Cholesterol: 27mg

Sodium: 40mg

Carbohydrates: 13g

Fiber: 2g

Phosphorus: 48mg

Potassium: 200mg

Protein: 1g

16. Zucchini Noodles with Spring Vegetables

Preparation Time: 20 minutes

Cooking Time: 10 minutes

Servings: 6

Ingredients:

6 zucchinis, cut into long noodles

1 cup of halved snow peas

1 cup (3-inch pieces) of asparagus

1 tablespoon of olive oil

1 teaspoon of minced fresh garlic

1 tablespoon of freshly squeezed lemon juice

1 cup of shredded fresh spinach

¾ cup of halved cherry tomatoes

2 tablespoons of chopped fresh basil leaves

Directions:

Fill a medium saucepan with water, put over medium-high heat, and bring to a boil.

Reduce the heat to medium, and blanch the zucchini ribbons, snow peas, and asparagus by submerging them in the water for 1 minute. Drain and rinse immediately under cold water.

Pat the vegetables dry with paper towels, and transfer to a large bowl.

Place a medium skillet, and

add the olive oil. Add the garlic, and sauté until tender, about 3 minutes.

Add the lemon juice and spinach, and sauté until the spinach is wilted about 3 minutes.

Add the zucchini mixture, the cherry tomatoes, and basil and toss until well combined.

Serve immediately.

Nutrition:

Calories: 52

Total fat: 2g

Saturated fat: 0g

Cholesterol: 0mg

Sodium: 7mg

Carbohydrates: 4g

Fiber: 1g

Phosphorus: 40mg

Potassium: 197mg

Protein: 2g

Chapter 3. Lunch

17.   Deviled Eggs

Preparation Time: 10 minutes

Cooking time: 45 minutes

Servings: 1 serving

Ingredients:

Hard-boiled egg (1)

Pimentos (1 teaspoon)

Mayonnaise (1 tablespoon)

Dry mustard (¼ teaspoon)

Black pepper (¼ teaspoon)

paprika (for garnishing)

Directions:

1. Cut the egg into two halves and remove the yolk.

2. Mix the pimentos, egg yolk, mayonnaise, dry mustard, and black pepper in a bowl.

3. Spoon the mixture into the halved egg whites in equal parts.

4. Sprinkle eggs with paprika, if you like.

Nutrition:

For one serving per recipe

Calories   116

Carbohydrates.   4 g

Phosphorus.   95 mg

Potassium.   83 mg

Protein.   7 g

Sodium.   78 mg

18.   Turkey and Noodles

Preparation Time: 10 minutes

Cooking time: 10 minutes

Servings: 8 servings

Ingredients:

- Dry elbow macaroni (2 cups)

- fresh lean ground turkey (2 pounds)

- Olive or vegetable oil (1 tablespoon)

- chopped green onions, (½ cup)

- chopped green pepper (½ cup)

- 14-ounce canned, regular diced tomatoes (1)

- black pepper (1 teaspoon)

- Italian seasoning (1 tablespoon)

Directions:

1. Transfer 4 cups of boiling water in a medium boiler and cook the macaroni for about 5 minutes or until tender.

2. Then drain the water and keep aside.

3. Heat the vegetable oil in a big fry pan over medium heat. Add the ground turkey to the oil and cook until its properly done while you stir occasionally.

4. Throw in the cooked macaroni, green peppers, onions, diced tomatoes, black pepper, and Italian seasoning. Mix well.

5. Serve warm.

Nutrition:

Calories. 273

Protein. 33 g

Carbohydrates. 22 g

Dietary fiber.   2 g

Sodium.   188 mg

Potassium.   533 mg

Phosphorus.   296 mg

19.   Eggplant Casserole

Preparation Time: 10 minutes

Cooking time: 45 minutes

Servings: 2 servings

Ingredients:

- Large eggplant (1)

- Lean ground turkey or beef (1 pound)

- Vegetable oil - 2 tablespoons (chopped)

- Plain bread crumbs (2 cups)

- green pepper - ½ cup (Chopped)

- onion - ½ cup (Chopped)

- large egg – 1 (slightly beaten)

- Red pepper - ½ teaspoon (optional)

Directions:

1. Preheat your oven to 350 degrees.

2. Boil the eggplant until it is tender, then drain and mash it

3. Heat the oil, then add the ground meat, onion, and green pepper. Sauté until cooked.

4. Add the bread crumbs, eggplant, and egg. Mix well.

5. Add red pepper to taste, if you want.

6. Place in a casserole dish and bake for approximately 45 minutes.

7. Serve warm

Nutrition:

Calories.   240

Carbohydrates.   5 g

Dietary fibers.   4 g

Protein.   15 g

Sodium.   263 mg

Chapter 4.Fish and Seafood

20.   Thai Spiced Halibut

Preparation Time: 5 minutes

Cooking Time: 20 minutes

Servings: 2 servings

Ingredients:

- 2 tablespoons coconut oil

- 1 cup white rice

- ¼ teaspoon black pepper

- ½ diced red chili

- 1 tablespoon fresh basil

- 2 pressed garlic cloves

- 4 oz. halibut fillet

- 1 halved lime

- 2 sliced green onions

- 1 lime leaf

Directions:

1. Preheat oven to 400°F/Gas Mark 5.

2. Add half of the ingredients into baking paper and fold into a parcel.

3. Repeat for your second parcel.

4. Add to the oven for 15-20 minutes or until fish is thoroughly cooked through.

5. Serve with cooked rice.

Nutrition: Calories 311, Protein 16 g, Carbohydrates 17 g, Fat 15 g, Sodium (Na) 31 mg, Potassium (K) 418 mg, Phosphorus 257 mg

21. Homemade Tuna Niçoise

Preparation Time: 5 minutes

Cooking Time: 10 minutes

Servings: 2 servings

Ingredients:

- 1 egg

- ½ cup green beans

- ¼ sliced cucumber

- 1 juiced lemon

- 1 teaspoon black pepper

- ¼ sliced red onion

- 1 tablespoon olive oil

- 1 tablespoon capers

- 4 oz. drained canned tuna

- 4 iceberg lettuce leaves

- 1 teaspoon chopped fresh cilantro

Directions:

1. Prepare the salad by washing and slicing the lettuce, cucumber, and onion.

2. Add to a salad bowl.

3. Mix 1 tablespoon oil with the lemon juice, cilantro, and capers for a salad dressing. Set aside.

4. Boil a pan of water on high heat then lower to simmer and add the egg for 6 minutes. (Steam the green beans over the same pan in a steamer/colander for the 6 minutes).

5. Remove the egg and rinse under cold water.

6. Peel before slicing in half.

7. Mix the tuna, salad, and dressing together in a salad bowl.

8. Toss to coat.

9. Top with the egg and serve with a sprinkle of black pepper.

Nutrition: Calories 199, Protein 19 g, Carbohydrates 7 g, Fat 8 g, Sodium (Na) 466 mg, Potassium (K) 251 mg, Phosphorus 211 mg

22.   Monk-Fish Curry

Preparation Time: 5 minutes

Cooking Time: 20 minutes

Servings: 2 servings

Ingredients:

- 1 garlic clove

- 3 finely chopped green onions

- 1 teaspoon grated ginger

- 1 cup water.

- 2 teaspoons chopped fresh basil

- 1 cup cooked rice noodles

- 1 tablespoon coconut oil

- ½ sliced red chili

- 4 oz. Monkfish fillet

- ½ finely sliced stick lemongrass

- 2 tablespoons chopped shallots

Directions:

1. Slice the Monkfish into bite-size pieces.

2. Crush the basil, garlic, ginger, chili, and lemongrass to form a paste using a pestle and mortar,

3. Now add the water to the pan and bring to a boil.

4. Add the Monkfish, lower the heat and cover to simmer for 10 minutes or until cooked through.

5. Enjoy with rice noodles and scatter with green onions to serve.

Nutrition: Calories 249, Protein 12 g, Carbohydrates 30 g, Fat 10 g, Sodium (Na) 32 mg, Potassium (K) 398 mg, Phosphorus 190 mg

23. Oregon Tuna Patties

Preparation Time: 10 minutes
Cooking Time: 15 minutes
Servings: 4
Ingredients:

- 1 (14.75 ounce) can tuna

- 2 tablespoons butter

- 1 medium onion, chopped

- 2/3 cup graham cracker crumbs

- 2 egg whites, beaten

- 1/4 cup chopped fresh parsley

- 1 teaspoon dry mustard

- 3 tablespoons olive oil

Directions:

1. Drain the tuna, reserving 3/4 cup of the liquid. Flake the meat. Melt butter in a large skillet over medium- high heat. Add onion, and cook until tender.

2. In a medium bowl, combine the onions with the reserved tuna liquid, 1/3 of the graham cracker crumbs, egg whites, parsley, mustard and tuna. Mix until well blended, then shape into six patties. Coat patties in remaining cracker crumbs.

3. Heat olive in a large skillet over medium heat. Cook patties until browned, then carefully turn and brown on the other side.

Nutrition:

Calories 204, Total Fat 15.4g, Saturated Fat 4.4g, Cholesterol 74mg, Sodium 111mg, Total Carbohydrate 6.5g, Dietary Fiber 0.9g, Total Sugar 2g, Protein 10.5g, Calcium 21mg, Iron 1mg, Potassium 164mg, Phosphorus 106mg

24. Fish Chowder

Preparation Time: 20 minutes

Cooking Time: 40 minutes

Servings: 4

Ingredients:

- 2 tablespoons butter

- 2 cups chopped onion

- 4 fresh mushrooms, sliced

- 1 stalk celery, chopped

- 4 cups chicken stock

- 2 pounds' cod, diced into 1/2 inch cubes

- 1/2 cup all-purpose flour

- 1/8 teaspoon Mrs. Dash salt-free seasoning, or to taste

- Ground black pepper to taste

- 2 (12 fluid ounce) cans soy milk

Directions:

1. In a large stockpot, dissolve 2 tablespoons butter. Sauté onions, mushrooms and celery in butter until tender.

2. Add chicken stock simmer for 10 minutes.

3. Add cod, and simmer another 10 minutes.

4. Mix flour until smooth; stir into soup and simmer for 1 minute more. Season to taste with seasoning, and pepper. Remove from heat, and stir in soy milk.

Nutrition:

Calories 171, Total Fat 4.2g, Saturated Fat 2.1g, Cholesterol 32mg, Sodium 810mg, Total Carbohydrate 19.3g, Dietary Fiber 2g, Total Sugar 3.9g, Protein 14.1g, Calcium 41mg, Iron 2mg, Potassium 204mg, Phosphorus 106mg

25. Tuna Salad with Cranberries

Preparation Time: 10 minutes

Cooking Time: 00 min

Servings: 4

Ingredient:

- 4 cans solid white tuna packed in water

- 2 tablespoons mayonnaise

- 1/3 teaspoon dried dill weed

- 3 tablespoons dried cranberries

Directions:

1. Put the tuna in a bowl, and mash with a fork.

2. Mix in mayonnaise to evenly coat tuna. Mix in dill and cranberries.

Nutrition:

Calories 81, Total Fat 2.8g, Saturated Fat 0.5g, Cholesterol 15mg, Sodium 74mg, Total Carbohydrate 2.3g, Dietary Fiber 0.2g, Total Sugar 0.7g, Protein 10.9g, Calcium 8mg, Iron 1mg, Potassium 113mg, Phosphorus 95mg

26. Zucchini Cups with Dill Cream and Smoked Tuna

Preparation Time: 15 minutes
Cooking Time: 35 minutes
Servings: 4

Ingredients:

- 1 1/3 large Zucchini
- 4 ounces' cream cheese, softened
- 2 tablespoons chopped fresh dill
- 1 teaspoon lemon zest
- 1/2 teaspoon fresh lemon juice
- 1/4 teaspoon ground black pepper
- 4 ounces smoked tuna, cut into 2-inch strips

Directions:

1. Trim ends from Zucchini and cut crosswise into 24 (3/4-inch-thick) rounds.

2. Scoop a 1/2-inch-deep depression from one side of each round with a small melon-baller, forming little cups.

3. Mix cream cheese, chopped dill, lemon zest, lemon juice, and black pepper together in a bowl. Spoon 1/2 teaspoon cheese mixture into each Zucchini cup. Top each cup with 1 tuna strip.

Nutrition:

Calories 51, Total Fat 3.8g, Saturated Fat 2.2g, Cholesterol 13mg, Sodium 219mg, Total Carbohydrate 1.8g, Dietary Fiber 0.3g, Total Sugar 0.6g, Protein 2.8g, Calcium 24mg, Iron 1mg, Potassium 95mg, Phosphorus 40mg

Chapter 5 .Meat & Poultry Recipes

27. Chicken Satay with Peanut Sauce

Preparation Time: 2 hours

Cooking Time: 11 minutes

Servings: 6

Ingredients:

For the chicken

- ½ cup plain, unsweetened yogurt

- 2 garlic cloves, minced

- 1-inch piece ginger, minced

- 2 teaspoons curry powder

- 1-pound boneless, skinless chicken breast, cut into strips

- 1 teaspoon canola oil

For the peanut sauce

- ¾ cup smooth unsalted peanut butter

- 1 teaspoon soy sauce

- 1 tablespoon brown sugar

- Juice of 2 limes

- ½ teaspoon red chili flakes

- ¼ cup hot water

- Fresh cilantro leaves, chopped, for garnish

- Lime wedges, for garnish

Directions:

To make the chicken

1. In a small bowl, add the yogurt, garlic, ginger, and curry powder. Stir to mix. Add the chicken strips to the marinade. Cover and refrigerate for 2 hours.

2. Thread the chicken pieces onto skewers.

3. Brush a grill pan with the oil, and heat on medium-high. Cook the chicken skewers on each side for 3 to 5 minutes, until cooked through.

To make the peanut sauce

4. Using food processor, mix peanut butter, soy sauce, brown sugar, lime juice, red chili flakes, and hot water. Process until smooth. Transfer to a bowl, and sprinkle with the cilantro. Serve with the

chicken satay along with lime wedges for squeezing over the skewers.

Nutrition:

286 Calories

25g Protein

33mg Phosphorus

66mg Potassium

201mg Sodium

28.   Chicken Breast and Bok Choy in Parchment

Preparation Time: 10 minutes

Cooking Time: 30 minutes

Servings: 4

Ingredients:

- 1 tablespoon Dijon mustard

- 1 tablespoon extra-virgin olive oil

- 1 tablespoon chopped fresh thyme leaves

- 2 cups thinly sliced bok choy

- 2 carrots, julienned

- 1 small leek, thinly sliced

- 4 boneless, skinless chicken breasts

- Freshly ground black pepper

- 4 lemon slices

Directions:

1. Preheat the oven to 425°F.

2. Blend mustard, olive oil, and thyme.

3. Prepare four pieces of parchment paper by folding four 18-inch pieces in half and cutting them like you would to create a heart. Open each piece and lay flat.

4. In each piece of parchment, arrange ½ cup of bok choy, a small handful of carrots, and a few slices of leek. Place the chicken breast on top, and season with pepper.

5. Brush the marinade over the chicken breasts, and top each with a slice of lemon.

6. Fold the packets shut, and fold the paper along the edges to crease and seal the packages.

7. Cook for 20 minutes. Let rest for 5 minutes, and open carefully to serve.

Nutrition:

164 Calories

24g Protein

26mg Phosphorus

187mg Potassium

356mg Sodium:

29. One-Pan Curried Chicken Thighs and Cauliflower

Preparation Time: 2 hours

Cooking Time: 40 minutes

Servings: 6

Ingredients:

- 3 tablespoons curry powder

- ½ teaspoon ground cumin

- ¼ teaspoon paprika

- ½ teaspoon freshly ground black pepper, divided

- 6 bone-in chicken thighs

- 4 teaspoons extra-virgin olive oil, divided

- 1 cauliflower head, cut into florets

- ½ teaspoon dried oregano

- Juice of 2 limes

Directions:

1. Combine curry powder, cumin, paprika, and ¼ teaspoon of pepper.

2. Pour 2 teaspoons of olive oil over the chicken thighs, and sprinkle with the curry mixture. Cover, refrigerate, and marinate for at least 2 hours or up to overnight.

3. Set the oven to 400°F.

4. Mix cauliflower with the remaining 2 teaspoons of olive oil and the oregano. In 1 layer, spread the chicken and cauliflower on a baking sheet.

5. Bake for 41 minutes, stirring the cauliflower and flipping the chicken pieces once during cooking.

6. Topped with the lime juice and serve.

Nutrition:

175 Calories

16g Protein

152mg Phosphorus

486mg Potassium

77mg Sodium

30. Asian-Style Pan-Fried Chicken

Preparation Time: 20 minutes

Cooking Time: 25 minutes

Servings: 4

Ingredients:

- 12 ounces boneless, skinless chicken thighs, fat removed, cut into 2 or 3 pieces each

- 1 teaspoon low-sodium soy sauce

- 1 teaspoon dry rice wine

- 1-inch piece ginger, minced

- ½ cup cornstarch

- 3 teaspoons canola oil, divided

- 1 lemon, cut into wedges

Directions:

1. In a medium bowl, combine the chicken, soy sauce, rice wine, and ginger. Toss and let sit for 15 minutes.

2. Toss the chicken again, and drain the liquid from the bowl. Simultaneously, dip the chicken pieces in the cornstarch to coat.

3. In a medium skillet over medium-high heat, heat 1½ teaspoons of oil. Add half of the chicken to the pan, and cook until golden brown on one side, about 3 to 5 minutes. Flip, and continue to cook on the opposite side, until the chicken is cooked through and is golden brown. Situate chicken to a plate lined with paper towels to cool. Add the remaining 1½ teaspoons of oil, and repeat the cooking process with the remaining chicken thighs.

4. Serve garnished with lemon wedges.

Nutrition:

198 Calories

17g Protein

148mg Phosphorus

218mg Potassium

119mg Sodium

31.   Chicken, Pasta, and Broccoli Bake

Preparation Time: 5 minutes

Cooking Time: 30 minutes

Servings: 6

Ingredients:

- 8 ounces' egg noodles

- 1 (10-ounce) package broccoli florets

- 2 tablespoons butter

- ½ sweet onion, chopped

- ¼ cup all-purpose flour

- 1½ cups Simple Chicken Broth or low-sodium store-bought chicken stock

- Freshly ground black pepper

- ¾ cup Homemade Rice Milk or unsweetened store-bought rice milk

- 3 cups shredded cooked chicken breast

- ¼ cup shredded Cheddar cheese

Directions:

1. Preheat the oven to 350°F. Grease a 2-quart dish.

2. Boil water. Add the egg noodles and cook for 5 minutes. Add the broccoli and continue to cook for 3 to 5 more minutes, until the noodles are tender and the broccoli is just fork-tender. Drain and set aside.

3. With a medium saucepan over medium-high heat, heat the butter. Add the onion and cook for 3 to 5 minutes, until it begins to soften. Add the flour and stir until evenly mixed. Add the broth and season with pepper. Simmer for 5 minutes, until it begins to thicken. Add the rice milk and cook until heated through.

4. Toss the sauce with the broccoli, noodles, and cooked chicken, and transfer to the prepared baking dish. Top with the Cheddar cheese.

5. Bake for 20 minutes, uncovered, until browned and bubbly.

Nutrition:

351 Calories

24g Protein

271mg Phosphorus

402mg Potassium

152mg Sodium

Chapter 6. Soup, Salad, Snacks & Light Meals Recipes

32.   Cabbage Stew

Preparation Time: 20 minutes

Cooking Time: 35 minutes

Servings: 6

Ingredients:

Unsalted butter – 1 tsp.

Large sweet onion - ½, chopped

Minced garlic – 1 tsp.

Shredded green cabbage – 6 cups

Celery stalks - 3, chopped with leafy tops

Scallion – 1, both green and white parts, chopped

Chopped fresh parsley – 2 Tbsps.

Freshly squeezed lemon juice – 2 Tbsps.

Chopped fresh thyme – 1 Tbsp.

Chopped savory – 1 tsp.

Chopped fresh oregano – 1 tsp.

Water

Fresh green beans – 1 cup, cut into 1-inch pieces

Ground black pepper

Directions:

Melt the butter in a pot.

Sauté the onion and garlic in the melted butter for 3 minutes, or until the vegetables are softened.

Add the celery, cabbage, scallion, parsley, lemon juice, thyme, savory, and oregano to the pot, add enough water to cover the vegetables by 4 inches.

Bring the soup to a boil.

Lessen the heat to low and simmer the soup for 25 minutes or until the vegetables are tender.

Season with pepper.

Nutrition:

Calories: 33

Fat: 1g

Carb: 6g

Phosphorus: 29mg

Potassium: 187mg

Sodium: 20mg

Protein: 1g

33.   Eggplant and Red Pepper Soup

Preparation Time: 20 minutes

Cooking Time: 40 minutes

Servings: 6

Ingredients:

Sweet onion – 1 small, cut into quarters

Small red bell peppers – 2, halved

Cubed eggplant – 2 cups

Garlic – 2 cloves, crushed

Olive oil – 1 Tbsp.

Chicken stock – 1 cup

Water

Chopped fresh basil – ¼ cup

Ground black pepper

Directions:

Preheat the oven to 350F.

Put the onions, red peppers, eggplant, and garlic in a baking dish.

Drizzle the vegetables with the olive oil.

Cook the vegetables for 30 minutes or until they are slightly charred and soft.

Cool the vegetables slightly and remove the skin from the peppers.

Puree the vegetables with a hand mixer (with the chicken stock).

Transfer the soup to a medium pot and add enough water to reach the desired thickness.

Heat the soup to a simmer and add the basil.

Season with pepper and serve.

Nutrition:

Calories: 61

Fat: 2g

Carb: 9g

Phosphorus: 33mg

Potassium: 198mg

Sodium: 98mg

Protein: 2g

34.   Kale Chips

Preparation Time: 20 minutes

Cooking Time: 25 minutes

Servings: 6

Ingredients:

Kale – 2 cups

Olive oil – 2 tsp.

Chili powder – ¼ tsp.

Pinch cayenne pepper

Directions:

Preheat the oven to 300F.

Get rid of the stems from the kale and tear the leaves into 2-inch pieces.

Wash the kale and dry it completely.

Handover the kale to a large bowl and drizzle with olive oil.

Use your hands to toss the kale with oil, taking care to coat each leaf evenly.

Season the kale with chili powder and cayenne pepper and toss to combine thoroughly.

Spread the seasoned kale in a single layer on each baking sheet. Do not overlap the leaves.

Bake the kale, rotating the pans once, for 20 to 25 minutes until it is crisp and dry.

Take out the oven trays and allow the chips to cool on the trays for 5 minutes.

Serve.

Nutrition:

Calories: 24

Fat: 2g

Carb: 2g

Phosphorus: 21mg

Potassium: 111mg

Sodium: 13mg

Protein: 1g

35.   Tortilla Chips

Preparation Time: 15 minutes

Cooking Time: 10 minutes

Servings: 6

Ingredients:

- Granulated sugar – 2 tsps.

- Ground cinnamon – ½ tsp.

- Pinch ground nutmeg

- Flour tortillas – 3 (6-inch)

- Cooking spray

Directions:

1. Preheat the oven to 350F.

2. Line a baking sheet with parchment paper.

3. Mix the sugar, cinnamon, and nutmeg.

4. Lay the tortillas on a clean work surface and spray both sides of each lightly with cooking spray.

5. Sprinkle the cinnamon sugar evenly over both sides of each tortilla.

6. Cut the tortillas into 16 wedges each and place them on the baking sheet.

7. Bake the tortilla wedges, turning once, for about 10 minutes or until crisp.

8. Cool the chips serve.

Nutrition:

Calories: 51

Fat: 1g

Carb: 9g

Phosphorus: 29mg

Potassium: 24mg

Sodium:103 mg

Protein: 1g

Chapter 7. Snacks

36.   Crunchy Chicken Nuggets

Preparation time: 25min

Cooking Time: 35min

Servings: 4

Ingredients:

- 2 - egg whites
- 1 - tablespoon water
- 2 ½ - cups ready-to-eat crispy rice cereal
- 1 ½ - teaspoons paprika
- ¼ - teaspoon seasoning salt
- ⅛ - teaspoon garlic powder
- ⅛ - teaspoon onion powder
- 1 - pound boneless, skinless chicken breasts
- 1 - tablespoon butter or margarine, melted
- 1 - tablespoon reduced-fat ranch dressing

Directions:

1. In a shallow dish join egg whites and water.
2. An enormous sheet of wax paper consolidates fresh rice oat, paprika, flavoring salt, garlic powder, and onion powder.
3. Cut chicken into 1 ½" pieces.
4. Plunge chicken into egg white blend, covering all sides. Come in grain blend.

5. A spot in a solitary layer on ungreased heating sheet. Shower with softened margarine.

6. Heat at 450°F for around 12 minutes or until never again pink in focus.

7. Serve warm with plunging sauce.

Nutrition: Calories 122, Fat 4g, Protein 14g, Carb 8g

37. Almond cranberry stuffed celery sticks

Preparation time: 5 Mins

Cooking Time: 5 Mins

Servings: 4

Ingredients:

- 4 Medium cut celery ribs
- 4 tablespoons of mixed berry whipped cream cheese
- 24 dried cranberries
- 11 whole dry roasted and unsalted whole almonds

Directions:

1. Start by trimming the ends of the celery ribs; then fill each of the ribs with 1 tablespoon of whipped cream cheese

2. Fill each of the celery ribs with 1 tablespoon of the whipped cream cheese.

3. Cut each of the celery ribs into 3 to 4 pieces according to the length

4. Top each of the celery rib pieces with 2 dried cranberries and 1 almond.

5. Refrigerate for about 10 minutes; then serve and enjoy your snack!

Nutrition:

Calories: 72, Fats: 5.6g, Carbs: 3g, Fiber: 0.8g, Potassium: 138mg, Sodium: 65mg, Phosphorous: 33mg, Protein 2g

38.   Cucumber and Onion dip

Preparation time: 3 Mins

Cooking Time: 4 Mins

Servings: 4

Ingredients:

- 8 Ounces of cream cheese
- 1 Medium cucumber
- 1 teaspoon of onion
- 1 tablespoon of lemon juice
- 1/8 teaspoon of green food coloring

Directions:

1. Set the cream cheese out of the refrigerator to soften.

2. Peel the cucumber, seed it; then and finely mince it

3. Mix the cream cheese, the onion, the lemon juice and the green food coloring in a medium bowl and blend your ingredients until it becomes smooth.

4. Fold the cucumber into the mixture until it becomes evenly blended.

Nutrition:

Calories: 120, Fats: 9g, Carbs: 8.5g, Fiber: 1.1g, Potassium: 138mg, Sodium: 65mg, Phosphorous: 33mg, Protein 1.3g

Chapter 8. Desserts

39.   Christmas Cake

Preparation Time: 17 minutes

Cooking Time: 31 minutes

Servings: 8

Ingredients:

- 200g glace cherries (Halved)

- 200g mixed peel

- 100g tinned peaches (Drained and roughly chopped)

- 100g tinned pineapple (Drained and roughly chopped)

- 2eggs (Beaten)

- 1 tablespoon brandy

- 250g plain flour

- 150g self-rising flour

- 200g unsalted butter

- 150g caster sugar

- 1 tablespoon nutmeg

- 2 tablespoons mixed spice

Directions:

1. Prepare the oven to 150°C/300°F/Gas 4.

2. Grease and line a 7in baking tin.

3. Cream butter and sugar until light and fluffy. Sieve the flour and spices together. Add the eggs and flour alternately to the creamed mixture, mixing well after each addition. Stir in the fruit, peel and brandy. Turn into the tin and cook for 3hours.

4. Ice when cool with white icing but avoid marzipan which is high in phosphate.

Nutrition:

584 calories

11g protein

99mg potassium

179mg sodium

40.   Gingerbread Yule Log

Preparation Time: 8 minutes

Cooking Time: 38 minutes

Servings: 6

Ingredients:

- 50g butter (Plus extra for greasing)

- 50g treacle

- 50g golden syrup

- 2 balls of stem ginger (Finely grated)

- 2 tablespoons of the syrup of the grated ginger

- 4 large eggs

- 100g dark muscovite sugar (Plus extra for dusting)

- 100g plain flour

- ½ tsp. baking powder

- 2 tablespoons ground ginger

- ½ tsp. ground cinnamon

For the icing
- 200g butter (Softened)

- 250g icing sugar

- 2tsp. vanilla extract

- 3tbsp. ginger syrup from the stem ginger jar

Directions:
1. Heat oven to 190C. Grease and prep 20 x 30cm Swiss roll tin with baking parchment, then grease

the parchment a little too. Situate treacle, syrup, butter and stem ginger in a pan, until melted and stir to combine, then set aside to cool a little.

2. Whisk eggs and sugar using an electric hand whisk until light, mousse-like and doubled in size – this will take about 10 minutes. Sift the flour, spices and baking powder then pour the melted butter mixture around the sides of the bowl. Once mixed, pour the mixture into the Swiss roll tin and ease it into the corners. Bake for 12 minutes

3. While cooking, spread a sheet of baking parchment big enough to fit the cake on your work surface and dust with a little sugar. Once done cooking, tip the cake directly onto the parchment. Put a line about 2cm from one of the shorter ends, making sure you don't cut all the way through. Lightly roll up from this end, rolling the parchment between the layers. Set aside to cool like this on a wire rack to help set the shape.

4. To make the icing, whisk the ingredients until smooth. Pour into a piping bag fitted with a large round nozzle or use a plastic sandwich bag and snip off one corner to make a hole about 1cm wide. Unroll the sponge and drizzle the surface with 2

tbsp. ginger syrup. Pipe a layer of ginger buttercream over the inside of the roll, then use the paper underneath to help tightly re-roll into a roulade. Slice off both ends for a neat finish. The butcher can be frozen. Defrost at room temperature before continuing.

5. Place the Bache on a serving plate or board. With the remaining icing use to pipe a thick layer over the sponge, zigzagging backwards and forwards to create a tight concertina pattern. Decorate with white pearl sprinkles, if you like.

Nutrition:

474 calories

17g protein

42mg potassium

161mg sodium

41.   Syrup Sponge Pudding

Preparation Time: 7 minutes

Cooking Time: 38 minutes

Servings: 4

Ingredients:

- 100g softened unsalted butter

- 100g caster sugar

- 2eggs

- 100g self-rising flour

- 6 tablespoons golden syrup

Directions:

1. Cream the butter and sugar together in a bowl or food processor.

2. Add one egg and mix carefully with a spoon of flour to prevent curdling. Add the other egg and mix well.

3. Fold in the flour.

4. Measure the syrup into a buttered pudding dish. Spoon the cake mixture on top of the syrup.

5. Cover with buttered foil with a fold to allow for expansion.

6. Bake at 200°C (180°C Fan)/400°F/Gas 6 for 35-40 minutes until a skewer comes out clean.

Nutrition:

364 calories

9g protein

79mg potassium

140mg sodium

42. Blackberry Lemon Muffins

Preparation Time: 11 minutes

Cooking Time: 31 minutes

Servings: 6

Ingredients:

- 1 cup All-purpose flour

- ¾ cup Whole Wheat flour

- ½ cup granulated sugar

- 2 tablespoons Baking powder

- ½ tablespoon Baking soda

- 1 tablespoon Grated lemon or orange peel

- 1 and a ½ cups Coffee Rich

- ½ cup Margarine (Melted)

- 2 egg whites

- 1 cup Fresh or frozen unsweetened blackberries

Directions:

1. Preheat oven to 375 F.

2. Incorporate flours with sugar, baking powder, baking soda, and lemon peel.

3. In a medium bowl, whisk Coffee Rich® with margarine and egg whites until blended. Stir Coffee Rich® mixture into flour mixture just until combined.

4. Fold in blackberries.

5. Scoop batter into lightly greased, paper lined muffin tins.

6. Bake for 21 minutes.

Nutrition:

564 calories

13g protein

40mg potassium

161mg sodium

43.   Quick Canned Pear Dessert

Preparation Time: 9 minutes

Cooking Time: 15 minutes

Servings: 4

Ingredients:

- cup ungifted flour

- ¼ cup Sugar

- ¼ cup unsalted Butter or Margarine

- 3 cups canned pears

- 2 tablespoons Lemon juice

- ¼ cup Sherry

- ¼ tsp. Nutmeg

Directions:

1. Preheat oven to 350 0F

2. In a medium bowl, mix flour and sugar together.

3. Using two knives or pastry blender, slice margarine or butter and flour until mixture is crumbly.

4. Set aside. Drain canned pears.

5. Place sliced pears into a well-greased 9-inch pie plate.

6. Drizzle fruit with lemon juice, sherry and nutmeg; dust flour mixture over top.

7. Bake for 15 minutes

Nutrition:

399 calories

16g protein

31mg potassium

144mg sodium

44. Renal Friendly Bran Muffins

Preparation Time: 7 minutes

Cooking Time: 36 minutes

Servings: 6

Ingredients:

- ¼ cup oil

- 1 egg

- 1 tsp. vanilla

- 1/3 cup honey

- 1 cup applesauce or crushed pineapple (Drained)

- 1 cup white flour

- 1 cup wheat bran

- 1 and a ½ tsp. baking soda

- ¼ tsp. cream of tartar

Directions:

1. Prep oven to 400°F and slightly grease muffin tins

2. Combine together, spoon into muffin tins and bake immediately.

3. Baking soda and cream of tartar will only rise once so do not delay getting the muffins into the oven.

4. Bake for 18 minutes.

Nutrition:

355 calories

17g protein

69mg potassium

147mg sodium

45.   Finland's Stripped Cake

Preparation Time: 14 minutes

Cooking Time: 32 minutes

Servings: 8

Ingredients:

- 3 cups ungifted all-purpose flour

- 1 cup sugar

- 1 teaspoon baking powder

- 1 cup (½ pound) butter or margarine (Softened)

- 2 whole eggs plus 1 egg white

- ½ teaspoon vanilla

- 1 cup jelly or jam (Plum, blackberry, or raspberry jelly, or apricot jam)

- 2 tablespoons sugar

Directions:

1. Heat oven to 375°F.

2. In a large bowl, combine flour, sugar, and baking powder.

3. Blend in butter with finger tips or pastry blender until mixture resembles cornmeal.

4. Add eggs, egg white and vanilla; work into stiff dough.

5. Divide dough into two balls, one twice the size of the other. On a heavily floured board (¼ to ½ cup flour), roll out the larger ball to 1/8" thickness.

6. Place rolled dough in a cookie pan (11" x 15 ½"), smoothing out to edges and patching corners. Spread jelly over the top.

7. Roll out remaining dough to 1/8" thickness and cut into ½ " wide strips; place strips diagonally across the jelly, ½" apart. Sprinkle sugar over the top. Place in oven.

8. When edges start to brown (about 20 minutes), take pan from the oven, cut off and remove about a 3" strip all around the edges. Return pan to oven, remove after 10 minutes.

9. Cut into 1" x 2" rectangles. Makes 7 dozen cookies.

Nutrition:

484 calories

9g protein

59mg potassium

166mg sodium

46.   Lemon Pastry Squares

Preparation Time: 12 minutes

Cooking Time: 29 minutes

Servings: 5

Ingredients:

For crust layer

- ¼ cup powdered sugar

- 1/8 Teaspoon salt

- 1 cup all-purpose flour

- ½ cup unsalted butter

For filling layer

- 1 cup granulated sugar

- ½ teaspoon baking powder

- 1/8 Teaspoon salt

- 2 eggs (Slightly beaten)

- 2 tablespoons fresh lemon juice

- Zest from one lemon

For icing layer

- 2 tablespoons fresh lemon juice

- ¾ cup powdered sugar

- 1 tablespoon unsalted butter (Softened)

Directions:

For crust layer

1. Mix all ingredients together.

2. Press into ungreased 8" square pan

3. Bake at 350° F for 15 minutes.

4. Remove from oven and spread with the filling layer.

For filling layer

5. Mix all filling ingredients together.

6. Spread evenly on top of baked crust layer.

7. Return to oven, and bake an additional 20 minutes at 350°F.

8. Remove from oven and cool.

For icing layer

9. Mix all ingredients together.

10. When baked crust and filling are completely cool, spread icing over the top.

Nutrition:

364 calories

8g protein

49mg potassium

171mg sodium

47. Classic Lemon Pound Cake

Preparation Time: 9 minutes

Cooking Time: 22 minutes

Servings: 8

Ingredients:

- 2 cups butter or margarine

- 4 cups powdered sugar

- 2 tablespoons grated lemon rind

- 1 teaspoon lemon extract

- 6 eggs

- 3 ½ cups all-purpose flour (Sifted)

Directions:

1. Preheat oven to 350°F.

2. With an electric mixer on medium speed, beat butter for 3 minutes, or until light and fluffy.

3. Gradually add sugar and rind; cream thoroughly.

4. Add lemon extract and eggs, one at a time, mixing well after each addition.

5. Gradually add flour; mix well.

6. Pour into greased and floured 10" tube pan.

7. Bake 80 minutes.

8. Remove from pan and cool.

Nutrition:

474 calories

8g protein

49mg potassium

168mg sodium

48. Glazed Pineapple Cake

Preparation Time: 11 minutes

Cooking Time: 29 minutes

Servings: 6

Ingredients:

For cake

- 3cups sugar

- 1and a ½ cups butter

- 6whole eggs and 4 egg whites

- 1teaspoon vanilla extract

- 3cups all-purpose flour (Sifted)

- One 300g can crushed pineapple (drain and reserve juice)

For glaze

- 1 cup sugar

- 1 stick margarine (½ cup)

- Juice from pineapple

Directions:

1. Preheat oven to 350°F.

2. Beat together sugar and butter until smooth and creamy.

3. Add eggs and egg whites two at a time, mixing after each addition.

4. Add vanilla.

5. Add sifted flour and mix well.

6. Add drained, crushed pineapple.

7. Bake for 45 minutes to 1 hour.

8. In a medium saucepan, mix together ingredients for glaze. Stir frequently. Bring to a boil, until desired thickness is reached. Pour over top of cake while hot.

Nutrition:

514 calories

11g protein

47mg potassium

161mg sodium

49.   Cinnamon Pound Cake

Preparation Time: 7 minutes

Cooking Time: 24 minutes

Servings: 5

Ingredients:

- 3 sticks butter or margarine

- ¼ teaspoons nutmeg powder

- 1 teaspoon Cinnamon powder

- 1 teaspoon vanilla extract

- 1-pound sifted powdered sugar

- 6eggs

- 3 cups all-purpose flour

- Powdered sugar (Garnish)

Directions:

1. Preheat oven to 325°F.

2. Beat butter in a huge bowl until softened.

3. Blend in nutmeg or mace and vanilla extract.

4. Gradually stir in powdered sugar.

5. Add eggs, one at a time, beating well after each addition.

6. Gradually stir in flour.

7. Grease only the bottom and lightly flour a 10" x 4" round tube pan. Do not grease the sides!

8. Bake for 1 hour and 20 minutes or until a cake tester inserted in the center comes out clean.

9. Allow cake to cool. Sprinkle with powdered sugar when cold.

Nutrition:

364 calories

13g protein

59mg potassium

129mg sodium

50.　Home Baked Simple Biscuits

Preparation Time: 9 minutes

Cooking Time: 32 minutes

Servings: 6

Ingredients:

- 2 cups all-purpose flour (Sifted)

- 3 teaspoons double acting baking powder

- 2 teaspoons sugar

- 1/3 Cup vegetable shortening

- ¼ cup 1% milk

- ½ cup water

Directions:

1. Pre-heat oven at 350°F. Sift dry ingredients into a bowl.

2. Cut in shortening until coarse crumbs form. Make a well in the mixture.

3. Pour milk and water into the well.

4. Stir quickly with a fork until dough follows fork around the bowl.

5. Dough should be soft. Turn dough onto lightly floured surface.

6. Knead gently 10-12 times. Roll or pat dough until ½" thick.

7. Dip a 2 ½" biscuit cutter into flour; then cut out 10 biscuits.

8. Bake biscuits on ungreased baking sheet for 12-15 minutes.

Nutrition:

374 calories

14g protein

49mg potassium

172mg sodium

Conclusion

Thank you for making it to the end. Patients who struggle with kidney health issues, going through kidney dialysis, and having renal impairments need to go through medical treatment and change their eating habit and lifestyle to make the situation better.

The first thing to changing your lifestyle is knowing how your kidney functions and how different foods can trigger different kidney function reactions. Certain nutrients affect your kidney directly. Nutrients like sodium, protein, phosphate, and potassium are the risky ones. You do not have to omit them altogether from your diet, but you need to limit or minimize their intake as much as possible. You cannot leave out essential nutrient like protein from your diet, but you need to count how much protein you are having per day. This is essential to keep balance in your muscles and maintaining a good functioning kidney.

A vast change in kidney patients is measuring how much fluid they are drinking. This is a crucial change in every kidney patient, and you must adapt to this new eating habit. Too much water or any other form of liquid can disrupt your kidney function. How much fluid you can consume depends on the condition of your kidney. Most people assign separate bottles for them to measure how much they have drunk and how much more they can drink throughout the day.

Like all other body parts, human kidneys also need much care and attention to work effectively. It takes a few simple and consistent measures to keep them healthy. Remember that no medicine can guarantee good health, but only a better lifestyle can do so. Here are a few of the practices that can keep your kidneys stay healthy for life.

Active lifestyle an active routine is imperative for good health. This may include regular exercise, yoga, or sports and physical activities. The more you move your body, the better its metabolism gets. The loss of water is compensated by drinking more water, and that constantly drains all the toxins and waste from the kidneys. It also helps control blood pressure, cholesterol levels, and diabetes, which indirectly prevents kidney disease.

Control blood pressure Constant high blood pressure may cause glomerular damage. It is one of the leading causes, and every 3 out of 5 people suffering from hypertension also suffer from kidney problems. The normal human blood pressure is below 120/80 mmHg. When there is a constant increase of this pressure up to 140/100mmHg or more it should be immediately put under control. This can be done by minimizing the salt intake, controlling the cholesterol level and taking care of cardiac health.

Hydration drinking more water and salt-free fluids proves to be the life support for kidneys. Water and fluids dilute the blood consistency and lead to more urination; this will release most of the excretions out of the body without much difficulty. It is the lack of water which strains the kidneys and often hinders the glomerular filtration. Water is the best option, but fresh fruit juices with no salt and preservatives are also vital for kidney health. Keep all of them in constant daily use.

Dietary changes there are certain food items which taken in excess can cause renal problems. In this regard, an extremely high protein diet, food rich in sodium, potassium, and phosphorous can be harmful. People suffering from early stages of renal disease should reduce their intake, whereas those facing critical stages of CKD should avoid their use altogether. A well-planned renal diet can prove to be significant in this regard. It effectively restricts all such food items from the diet and promotes the use of more fluids, water, organic fruits, and a low protein meal plan.

No smoking/alcohol Smoking and excessive use of alcohol are other names for intoxication. Intoxication is another major cause of kidney disease, or at least it aggravates the condition. Smoking and drinking alcohol indirectly pollute the blood and body tissues, which leads to progressive kidney damage. Begin by gradually reducing alcohol consumption and smoking down to a minimum.

Monitor the changes since the early signs of kidney disease are hardly detectable, it is important to keep track of the changes you witness in your body. Even the frequency of urination and loss of appetite are good enough reasons to be cautious and concerning. It is true that only a health expert can accurately diagnose the disease, but personal care and attention to minor changes is of key importance when it comes to CKD. I hope you have learned something!